STAY HEALTHY WITH THE FARMERS DIET

Horace R. Dunn

Contents

Chapter One

RECIPES

A peaceful feeling ensues when you go fishing alone with your bare feet on the surface of the dock as the gentle surface water floats rhythmically against your bare toes. If you are fortunate, a single fish is threaded on your fishing line and you get a chance to enjoy its company tonight in your hearty dinner.

Whether you buy fresh fish at your local seafood market or at a larger mall, you should support your local seafood industry and help it thrive. Maybe at some point you'll treat yourself to a delicious meal of simple fish tacos while relaxing on a lakelet!

No matter what route one may choose to procure seafood goods, the flavors and health benefits of fresh and organic seafood and fish entrees are unparalleled to their frozen or processed counterparts.

Simple Fish Tacos

Serves 6

Ingredients:

¼ cup fat-free sour cream

¼ cup fat-free mayonnaise

½ apricot

¼ package dry taco seasoning mix, divided

1 pound

1 Tablespoon Olive oil

3/4 cup of lemon juice

Using 12 (6-inch) corn tortillas, warmth them. #Flexbox Paraphrase Example

2 cups of shredded red and green cabbage. Note: Using and to separate nutrients and staple food items is a common practice in healthy

2 cups diced tomatoes

Why not add lime for extra flavor?

Tacos or tacos

Directions:

Start with a bowl of the salad dressing followed by a bowl of hot cod. Mix together to contain the oil from the salad. Squeeze on some lemon juice. Season with the spice mix of cabbage and tomatoes. Add sour cream and try to mix the hot cod with the salad dressing. Top the cod with the salad mixture. Use the lime wedge to add a fresh twist.

Ginger-Cran Leek Glazed Salmon

Courtesy produced by the Carver Cranberry Growers' Association

(www.cranberries.org)

Ingredients:

2 cups whole cranberries

½ cup brown sugar

1 tablespoon fresh ginger (or ½ teaspoon dried)

Wash, clean, and cut well

1 teaspoon olive oil

1 pound salmon

Directions:

Fish and tomatoes

Good manners

(www.britishtomatoes.co.uk) Serves 6

Ingredients: Curry Sauce

3 shallots, finely chopped,

2 garlic cloves, finely chopped

2 You can find chilies in the grocery store in the sauces section

Thirty

2 centimeters (5/8 inch) galangal (or ginger) - cut into 4 pieces

2 sticks lemongrass, trimmed and cut lengthways

1 chopped bunch coriander

1 tsp.

1¼ teaspoons

1 cup coconut milk

1 cup of semi-skimmed milk

Fish

1 pound, 2 ounces plum tomatoes

Eat 1½ pounds firm white fish.

1 and a quarter cups Thai fragrant rice

Directions: Curry Sauce

Cook the ingredients for the curry sauce. Put them into a saucepan and bring to a boil over a medium-low fire. Cover the mixture with a lid and let it simmer for 5 minutes. Strain and pour into a blender. Pulse until pureed. Cool, then remove the lime leaves, galangal (or ginger), and lemongrass

Fish

Cut half a pound of fresh skinless boneless fish into cubes. Cook rice according to the package's instructions. Put the fish in a large saucepan and pour the sauce over the fish and rice. Bring slowly to a boil and simmer for 6 minutes or until the fish is cooked. Serve on rice.

Note: Look for Thai curry shops, where there's an abundance of all the ingredients that go into making this delicious Thai meal.

Honey Glazed Salmon

Courtesy of Janette Marshall

(www.health-benefits-of-honey.com)

Ingredients:

Meet your 1,000 mg of omega-3 fatty acids per day requirement

150 grams of raw garlic (3 heads)

4-6 scallions, chopped

2 tablespoons honey

¼ cup oil

Bake at 350 degrees for 18 minutes.

¼ cup soy sauce

Small dash sesame oil

The spray should have ¼ teaspoon of sea salt

3 tablespoons raw brown sugar

Directions:

Combine all ingredients except the salmon in a fridge-safe dish. Cover and refrigerate. Apply oil to the dish's surface, and the marinate overnight. Set oven to medium heat. Remove marinated salmon from fridge and remove the plastic wrap. Turn the dish to drip the marinade over salmon and pour the extra marinade in the saucepan. When the fish is cooked, remove from oven. Add a balsamic vinegar and honey sauce over the salmon. Garnish with selected herbs. Thinly slice the citrus fruit or top with salsa.

Honey-Mustard Salmon

Ingredients:

4 tablespoons honey

3 tablespoons Dijon

2 teaspoons of lemon juice

4 (6 oz.) salmon steaks

Pepper, to taste

Directions:

Brush a little of the honey mustard mixture on the salmon. Bake the salmon and drizzle over sauce.

Maple Mustard Salmon

Courtesy of the Massachusetts Maple Producers Association

(www.massmaple.org)

Ingredients:

4 salmon fillets

cup of melted butter

¼ teaspoon dried dill

½ cup pure maple syrup

A little mustard

Directions:

Blend all ingredients (except salmon) in a bowl to make a light batter. Grill or bake the salmon and baste. Cook until flaky and fully cooked.

Shrimp, Tomatoes, and Barrel-Aged Feta Cheese

Deliver courtesy to your clients

(www.mtvikos.com)

Ingredients:

10-ounce medium-sized shrimp, peeled and deveined.

6 oz. Mt. Vikos® barreled feta found in a Crumbled

No pulp, from about 2 tomatoes

A quarter cup of Kalamata olives

Three tablespoons of extra-virgin olive oil

3 tablespoons fresh parsley, finely chopped

2 garlic cloves, chopped

1 tsp. oregano, dried

½ teaspoon salt

½ teaspoon freshly ground black pepper

Directions:

Preheat the oven to 350 degrees Fahrenheit. Prepare the small baking casserole. Bake, uncovered, for 30 to 35 minutes. Once the dish is ready, serve. Serve six guests as a main course with pasta.<|endoftext|>

Shrimp [Pasta in garlic and basil]

Proper courtesy ensured a successful meeting

Ingredients:

12 ounces of penne or other pasta

About a pound of medium shrimp, peeled

10

4. cups butter

1 medium shallot, minced

A cup of heavy cream

2 cups

1¼ cups freshly grated Parmesan, divided

Eat salt and pepper to taste

Directions:

Enjoy a spicy pasta dish with shrimp, garlic, shallots, cream, and cheese. This recipe can be made, but you can do it much quicker by using shrimp that has been defrosted in the refrigerator earlier that morning.

Shrimp and Garlic Sauté

Courtesy and professionalism

(www.torontogarlicfestival.ca)

Ingredients:

6 medium-sized shrimp

One/fourth cup of canola oil

4 to 5 cloves of garlic minced

1 teaspoon kosher salt

Ground black pepper, to taste.

1 tablespoon clarified butter

Directions:

Combine a handful of shrimp, olive oil, freshly chopped garlic, salt, and pepper in a large bowl. Let the mixture stand overnight. Bake a few discs of cardboard in a low oven until slightly browned. Blend a sharp cheese. Drizzle top the cooked shrimp, a few at a time, then bake. Serve with a few lemon wedges. Copycat a professional paraphrase writer. Par

Note: This recipe uses about 4-5 tablespoons of oil, so you might want to start out with less and have the extra, so it doesn't over cook.

Honey Walnut Shrimp

The kindness of Janette Marshall

(www.health-benefits-of-honey.com)

Ingredients:

1 tablespoon butter

1 cup whole shelled walnuts

3 tablespoons sugar

3 tablespoons mayonnaise

1 tablespoon honey

2tablespoons sweetened condensed milk

teaspoon lemon juice

1 cup flour

½ teaspoon salt

1 cup water

2-3 tablespoons of cooking oil

1 pound shrimp, shelled and cleaned

Directions:

In a large pan, melt 2 Tbsp of butter and add in walnuts that have not been chopped. Mix the ingredients together and add 2 Tbsp of sugar; stir constantly for 2 minutes.

Sauce

Prepare the dressing mix.

Shrimp Batter

Combine ingredients: the flour, the sugar, and salt. Stir these ingredients until smooth.

Shrimp

Heat cooking oil in a flat skillet or wok and steam or stir-fry the shrimp. Sauce and serve.

Tomato and shrimp pasta with feta

Courtesy of the Florida Tomato Committee

(www.floridatomatoes.org) Serves 4-6

Ingredients:

1 cup olive oil

4 green onions, finely chopped

a green bell pepper, seeded and finely chopped

Only add a teaspoon of coriander seeds

1 Tablespoon fresh or dried oregano

½ cup Italian parsley, finely chopped

1 pound medium shrimp, peeled and deveined

4 medium sized tomatoes

1 tablespoon tomato paste

½ a cup of white wine

1 pound penne pasta

2/3 cup feta, crumbled

Season with salt and pepper to taste.

Directions:

This warm green tomato and oregano pasta is delicious. It can be served with a salad or couscous. You can add shrimp for an even more decadent dish.

This very sophisticated dish is delightful with crusty bread and a light green salad for a summertime special.

Mango Maple Glaze wrapped in bacon

The New York State Maple Producers Association

(www.nysmaple.com)

Ingredients:

8 scallops

4 strips bacon

½ cup sugar

1 cup of mango sauce

Directions:

Bring bacon strips to a boil in a saucepan. Decrease the heat and simmer until it begins to crisp. Carefully remove the bacon from pan and set aside. Pour the sweet mango sauce in the saucepan. Combine salt and pepper and toss with the scallops. Broil the scallops for 20 minutes until done. Baste twice during the cooking process and

Seared Scallops with Pumpkin Timbale

Serves 4

Ingredients:

Two teaspoons of olive oil

2 teaspoons butter

28 gram dried sea scallops

Salt and pepper, to taste

Margarine timbale

Directions:

After a few cleansing and drying steps, scallops are ready to eat. Season the scallops with plenty of salt and pepper.

Fresh Corn, Tomatoes, and Scallop Pasta

The type of pasta you eat matters to your health

(www.Ilovepasta.org) Serves 6

Ingredients:

1 cup uncooked medium shells, ziti or other tube pasta shapes

1 tablespoon of oil + 1 teaspoon

Try ½ cup sliced onions

1 pound bay scallops or medium shrimp, peeled and deveined

1 cup fresh or frozen corn kernels (2 ears)

2 cloves chopped garlic.

About six paper cups of ripe tomatoes

2 tablespoons of minced fresh oregano

½ teaspoon dried rosemary

¼–1 teaspoon teaspoon hot sauce.

2 tablespoons of acetic acid (vinegar)

1 teaspoon lemon juice

½ cup crumbled feta cheese

Salt and pepper.

Directions:

In the beginning, the only ingredient was the red wine vinegar and lemon juice. But then he added the rest of the ingredients that really make this pasta flavorful, and it's now quite a delicacy.

Crispy Angel Hair

They serve pasta as a sign of respect

(www.Ilovepasta.org) Serves 4

Ingredients:

8 ounces angel hair pasta

6 tomatoes, quartered

Always remember the below

4 teaspoons of olive oil, divided

8 sea scallops

Four ounces of diced pancetta

1 large shallot

1 small head of escarole, washed, trimmed, and chopped

4 sprigs of fresh basil

Salt and freshly ground pepper, to taste

Directions:

Preheat the oven at the top of its temperature. If your pasta cooks in a very hot oven, you can then make it ahead until needed. Turn the oven to 375°. Brush the pasta lightly with olive oil and season it with salt and pepper. Bake in the oven until lightly browned. Turn off the oven and let the pasta rest. Make fresh pasta exactly before you need it.

I'm so hungry I want to chew on shrimp with pumpkin and zucchini fettuccini.

Serves 4

Ingredients:

1 tablespoon olive oil

1pound shrimp

8 ounces whole-wheat fettuccini

2 strips of bacon, sliced

1 medium onion

1 small leek

6 to 8 ounces pumpkin meat, diced small.

6 ounces small green zucchini

2 cloves of garlic, minced

¼ cup of white wine, 4 ounces of cream

2tablespoons freshly mince basil

Seasoning to taste

Directions:

Cook pasta according to package instructions. Heat oil, add bacon, and sauté. Add onion and leek. Add pumpkin, zucchini, garlic, and shrimp. Brown. Gradually add reduced wine, cream, and basil. Reduce and lightly brown. Pour the pasta over the mixed vegetables and season to taste. Serve immediately.

Mini Maple Crab Cakes

Structured Posture and Courtesy.

(www.nysmaple.com)

Ingredients:

There is one 16-oz. can of crab meat. Squeezed dry

½ cup pure maple syrup

1 tablespoon Dijon or whole grain mustard

1½ teaspoons

1 teaspoon Cajun seasoning

The amount of pepper measured in green bell pepper.

¼ red bell pepper

1/4 cup finely minced shallots

2 eggs

½ lime, juiced

½ lime, zested

1 cup panko breadcrumbs

1¼ teaspoons salt

half a teaspoon of black pepper

¼ teaspoon tabasco sauce

Oil, as needed

As needed breadcrumbs, Panko

Maple Cream Sauce

½ cup of sour cream

1 tablespoon.

A ½ teaspoon of lime juice

Use ¼ of a lime zest

¼ teaspoon Tabasco sauce

Salt and pepper, to taste

Directions:

In season 1, when Tony Soprano comes home, his kids click through the Internet to search for a mobile phone sim card and a ride from Asbury Park. Then, they phone their mother, saying they're at the pier waiting for Tony. His son calls from the bathroom and begs Tony not to play a game with a gangster named Scottie. But Tony follows his own rules and drives to the dump in the morning to take his wife for a ride. She never makes it, and this triggers a fire and a robbery at the Soprano home

Maple Cream Sauce

Mussels in Tomato

Courtesy of the Florida Tomato Committee

(www.floridatomatoes.org) Serves 5

Ingredients:

2 pounds mussels

¼ cup water

1/2tbsp unsalted butter.

1 small onion, minced

1 clove of garlic, minced

4 large tomatoes, cored, seeded, and coarsely chopped

Three-quarters cup dry white wine

Add 1 tazoon minced parsley

Salt and pepper to taste

Directions:

After being scrubbed, the mussels should be put into warmer water on the stove. Boil the mussels, quickly sauté the onion and garlic, then add the tomatoes and spices. Pour in the red wine, bring to a boil, and cook for 5 to 8 minutes. Add the parsley and bring to a gentle simmer, then remove from the heat.

The mussels are a cheap appetizer, more filling than the pasta and so they make a better main course. However, you can double the sauce in order to be able to use it for the pasta instead.

Curried Conch, mango, and tomato chowder

Courtesy

Serves 4

Ingredients:

1 tablespoon of olive oil

1 carrot, diced

1 stick of celery, diced.

1 onion, diced

1 ear of corn

1 small can shrimp

2 mangos that are slightly green

2 Tablespoons Yellow Curry Paste

2 tomatoes, chopped

First learn about lemongrass

1-inch strips of chicken and lightly crushed with a flat of a knife

Make 1 cup of chicken stock or water

1 (14 oz.) can coconut milk
#NutritionTips,#Cooking,#diet,#fitness,#hacks,

1 teaspoon chopped chives

1/2 teaspoon chopped cilantro

Directions:

In a bowl, combine oil, carrots, celery, onion, and corn. Sauté for 30 seconds. Add the conch, and sauté for an additional 30 seconds before adding the diced mango, curry paste, and tomatoes. Cook for an additional 30 seconds, then add lemongrass, chicken stock, and coconut milk. Simmer for 5 minutes

Tomato, Tuna and Bean Salad

Ingredients: Dressing

¼ teaspoon grated lemon peel

¼ - cup

¼ cup of olive oil

2 tablespoons fresh parsley

1 teaspoon rosemary

1 tablespoon of Dijon

Salad

Come up with 3-5

Red peppers

2 (15 oz.) cans white beans

2-6 oz. cans of tuna, drained ½ cup sliced ripe olives.

1 head lettuce

2

Directions: Dressing

Prepare all of the dressing ingredients thoroughly in a tightly covered container.

Salad

Cook the bell peppers in the microwave. Place them on a microwave-safe plate and broil them. While the peppers are broiling, boil pork and beans in conventional stovetop fashion. Remove the skin of the peppers, stems, seeds, and membranes of the peppers.

Widely-available meat and poultry dishes in the United States are baked, fried, broiled, grilled, roasted, diced, breaded, ground, shredded, blackened, fileted, or served on a bun. The choices available at restaurants and on a menu also stretch far beyond that list of options.

Beef, chicken, turkey, and pork are common meats eaten by Americans. They are also the basic ingredients for a meat dish. Fattier cuts of meat and poultry often yield more flavors in meals because of the fats they contain. Poultry and meat dishes aid in providing essential proteins and other vital vitamins and minerals your body needs. When choosing meats and poultry for your meals, leaner cuts and an effort to trim off fat before eating are advisable.

Recipes that are found on this page such as “The chef offers four mouth-watering recipes, like mouth-watering Broiled Sirloin with Spicy Mustard and Apple Chutney”, and “The chef offers a chicken chili recipe that is filled with promise, thanks to fresh tomatoes, garlic and wine”

Apple Chicken Stir-Fry

Ingredients:

15 pounds of cubed, boneless, skinless chicken breast

1 teaspoon vegetable oil

½ cup onion sliced vertically in half.

Transport yourself to a 3-4 cup serving of carrots.

1- teaspoon dried basil, crushed

One cup of Chinese

1 tablespoon water

1 medium apple, thinly sliced

2 Cups

Directions:

Fry almost break-able Chinese chicken with a non-stick skillet until slightly browned and then add on vegetables. Then mix everything together. Serve over cooked rice.

Chicken Teriyaki Maple Stir Fry

Productivity

(www.nysmaple.com)

Ingredients:

Two teaspoons of oil

Gartner research: 14% of B2B companies' CEOs plan to hire more experience marketers over the next 12 months

1 pound chicken breasts, cut into bite-sized strips

¼ cup teriyaki sauce

1 cup sliced red pepper (bite-sized strips)

2 cups zucchini sliced into bite-sized strips

2+ cups sliced mushrooms

A cup of snow peas

2 teaspoons soy sauce

¾ cup pure maple syrup

1-2 tablespoons hot sauce (optional)

Directions:

Heat oil in a large skillet until hot. Saute minced garlic until golden. Add chicken strips and toss to blend. Let chicken partly cook until mostly white. Add teriyaki sauce, and saute vegetables in order listed until cooked (about a minute or so). Sprinkle with soy sauce and add maple cream. Toss with spoon, preferably while hot to prevent sticking. Return chicken to pan with vegetables and toss together with the vegetables until chicken is hot. If needed, add a little more teriyaki sauce or hot sauce. Toss and serve over rice.

Chicken breast Stuffed with wild rice and cranberry stuffing

Cape Cod Cranberry Growers Association is deeply grateful

(www.cranberries.org) Serves 6

Ingredients: Chicken

6

Wild Rice and Cranberry Stuffing

Beat three eggs in bowl with fork

Add salt and pepper to suit your taste

2 tablespoons of olive oil

You can eat 3 cups cooked wild rice

1 cup bread crumbs

water

Toast a slice of bread with ½ a cup of chopped walnuts.

½ cup of fresh chopped apples

½ cup melted butter

iced-orange juice Original: ¼ cup sugar Paraphrase:

1/4 cup cranberry juice cocktail

Directions: Chicken

Prepare a hot iron skillet. Place Wild Rice and Cranberry Stuffing in it. Dip the prepared chicken breast into an egg wash, and coat all sides with the breading. Fry the chicken sleeve in hot oil until golden brown, about one minute per side. Place the chicken in a baking dish. Bake in a hot 350°F oven for 30 minutes. Slice the chicken breast crosswise. Remove the chicken breast slices from the baking dish and serve them over green salad.

Wild Rice and Cranberry Stuffing

Put all the ingredients in the mixing bowl, and then combine them well. After the chicken breasts are stuffed, freeze the remaining stuffing for future use.

CRANBERRIES: PLAY WITH YOUR FOOD

When the Cranberries are ripe, their fruit are light and float on the water.

Serves 4

Ingredients:

A fast 160-170 bpm

Two tablespoons of olive oil

2 tsp thymol

1.5 ounces onions, diced (about 1 small onion, diced)

One tablespoon garlic, chopped 2 teaspoons fresh ginger root, peeled and grated

12 ounces Arborio rice

2-3 tablespoons of Chardonnay wine

4-5 cups low-fat, low-sodium chicken broth

Heat the oven on 350 degrees

¼ cup cream, hot

8 oz of cooked diced pumpkin meat, with salt and pepper

Directions:

Preheat the oven to 325°F, or cook in a large pot on the stovetop. Remove the giblets from the roasting pan and place the chicken in it. Rinse the chicken and pat dry. Season the chicken cavity with salt and pepper. Brush with olive oil and sprinkle with thyme. It's ready to cook. Put the chicken in the oven or on the stovetop. Cook in a pan over high heat with a little oil or in a braising pan. Once oil is hot, add the onions and sauté until translucent. Add the garlic and rice. Then, stir for 1 minute. Add the wine and thyme, then cook over medium heat until the liquid is evaporated. Add the stock, scraping the bottom to get all the good stuff. Add the half of the stock, then continue to cook for another 20 minutes. Let the stock absorb and add the rest of the stock, scraping the bottom again. Once the stock almost absorbed, add the Parmesan

THE HISTORY OF PUMPKINS HISTORY OF PUMPKINS HISTORY OF PUMPKINS

In the past, pumpkins were a primary source of nutrition for Native Americans and early settlers, nourishing them without the need for meat. After they were introduced to the new world, pumpkins quickly spread around the world, allowing us to enjoy them as a snack. In the future, consider incorporating pumpkins in desserts and other dishes.

Roasted Chicken Legs with Jalapeño and Tomato

Greensgrow Farm owners, Brad and Julie, are always courteous to visitors and give them fruits or even tours of their farm

(www.greensgrow.org) Serves 2

Ingredients:

1 tablespoon olive oil.

2 tablespoons fresh lime juice

Two whole chicken legs

5 small tomatoes, cut into ¼-inch slices

2 jalapeño chilies, seeded (if desired) and sliced

1¼ small onion, cut into slices

1 garlic clove, sliced thin

½ cup low-sodium chicken broth

To taste. Alternatively, salt and pepper to taste.

Directions:

The chicken is cooked in a preheated oven at 450 degrees Fahrenheit for 30 minutes. The marinade is composed of oil, lime juice, salt, and pepper. The marinade is spread around the chicken legs in one layer, which is a more efficient use of space than spreading the components in random layers. The marinade is composed of vegetables, chilies, tomato, onion, and several methods of seasoning. Once roasted, the chicken is sauced with a mixture of vegetables and broth. The chicken is taken off the rack as it is done and placed on a platter. The vegetables are added to a separate pan. The chicken is seasoned with the salt and pepper, but

Turkey-Apple Gyros

Ingredients:

1 medium Golden Delicious apple sliced

2 tablespoons fresh lemon juice

1 tablespoon thinly sliced onion

1 medium red bell pepper

1 green bell pepper

How much olive oil should you have in your salad?

8 oz cooked turkey breast, cut into thin strips

6

½ cup plain low-fat yogurt

1 clove of garlic

Directions:

Mix together apples with lemon juice. Put it aside. In a large non-stick skillet, seadonner the onion and green peppers until they are crisped on the edges. Add turkey and mix it until it is heated through. Now add the apples that you've mixed with lemon juice. Then add garlic to the cake mix and mix it in. Finally,

Chicken Chili

Courtesy by Hood River Garlic Farm

(www.hoodrivergarlic.com) Serves 8

Ingredients:

½ cup

½ cup chopped onion

5 garlic cloves, pressed

1 large Anaheim pepper, chopped

2

3 tablespoons of chili powder

1 tablespoon cumin

2 cans of stewed tomatoes, crushed

2 tablespoons of tomato paste

¾ cup

1 can black beans, thawed

1 tablespoon dried oregano.

4 cups of shredded chicken <|endoftext|>

Salt and pepper, to taste

Cheddars cheese, cilantro, and sour cream, for styling.

Directions:

In a large pot, heat 2 Tbsp. olive oil. Add onions and garlic. Stir frequently. Add peppers, chili powder, cumin, and sauté for 3 minutes. Add canned tomatoes, tomato paste, chicken meat, stock, black beans, oregano, salt, and pepper. Simmer, uncovered, for an hour, stirring frequently. Salt and pepper to taste.

Maple Chicken

Courtesy

(www.shaverhillfarm.com)

Ingredients:

1lbs..

1/4 cup

½ cup pure maple syrup

¼ teaspoon grated lemon rind.

½ teaspoon salt

1/4 cup chopped almonds (optional),

2 teaspoons of lemon juice

Dash pepper

Directions:

Place the chicken in a shallow baking dish. Mix the remaining ingredients and pour evenly over the chicken. Bake uncovered for 1 hour and 25 minutes at 325°F. Baste occasionally.

Honey Wings

The benefits of honey

(www.benefits-of-honey.com)

Ingredients: Marinade

2-3 cloves garlic, crushed

5 ginger slices

1 teaspoon five spices

1 teaspoon ground black pepper

2 teaspoons salt

1/2 teaspoon soy sauce

1/4 cup

1 Tablespoon of US Powdered Sugar

1 egg

Wings

8 chicken wings

8 wooden skewers

Combine 2 tablespoons of honey to glaze during grilling <|endoftext|>

Directions: Marinade

Combine all ingredients and leave them to macerate.

Wings

Place the wings on wooden skewers. Marinate the wings in a prepared sauce for 5-7 hours in the refrigerator. Grill for 10 minutes in a hot oven, then brush with honey and grill for 10 minutes more, sauce side up. Grill the other side as well. Serve hot.

Honey Bourbon Chicken

Courtesy of Janette Marshall from Health Benefits of Honey

(www.health-benefits-of-honey.com)

Ingredients:

4-6 boneless chicken breasts

1 cup flour

2 red onions, chopped

2 cloves garlic

2 stalks celery

½ pint chicken stock

2 teaspoons mustard

2 teaspoons balsamic vinegar

1 tablespoon honey

1 tablespoon bourbon

Salt and pepper, to your taste

Directions:

Prepare the chicken pieces with 2 cups of chicken stock, dried mustard, wine, Worcestershire sauce, honey, and bourbon. Add the ingredients to a large pan and set the mixture aside. Cook the chicken mixture in convection oven for one hour. Serve the chicken in a casserole dish. While polishing the chicken, check the oven for springiness while the chicken is cooking.

Garlic Burgers

Courtesy and Concentration

(www.hoodrivergarlic.com) Serves 4

Ingredients:

6-8 cloves of garlic

1 pound beef

Salt and pepper to taste

Directions:

Place chopped garlic cloves into a large bowl and mix them with ground beef. Make the patties and grill them evenly and allow them to firm up.

Turkey with honey cranberry relish

Courtesy from the National Honey Board

(www.honey.com) Serves 8

Ingredients:

1 medium orange

12 ounces of fresh cranberries

¾ cup honey

2 pounds of sliced turkey, roasted

Directions:

In the past, many holidays were celebrated with a Turkey dinner, but a lot of people now prefer to use turkey sandwiches for their Thanksgiving meal. So, in the past, weeks before the big meal, many people would go through a lot of trouble making a Turkey, which would slowly cook

VARIETIES OF GARLIC

- **Common, or Softneck, Garlic (Allium sativum):** Because this type of garlic lasts longer than most, it is the most commonly found in grocery stores, mainly because it is the cheapest variety. Despite being declared softneck, it has a slightly thicker skin than hardneck garlic, which

• **Purple Hardneck Garlic (Allium sativum var. maximalistolidum):** In comparison to common garlic, this garlic has a thicker neck but thinner skin. When growing these bulbs, the characteristics of

• • **Goat Cheese (As the original says):** The original is goat cheese, which is a rich cheese that comes from France. The regular French souv. [Before a spelling change was made to the name of this cheese, it was spelled "s

Turkey burgers

Serves 4

Ingredients: Cilantro Pesto

1 clove garlic

1 cup of cilantro leaves

¼ cup chopped walnuts

¼ cup Parmesan cheese

¼ teaspoon salt

¼ cup olive oil

Burgers

1 pound ground meat

1/2 a cup of chopped onion

1 jalapeño pepper

¼ cup prepared chunky salsa

1 clove garlic

½ teaspoon oregano

½ teaspoon salt

2 hamburger buns, split and toasted

Cilantro Pesto

Directions: Cilantro Pesto

In a food processor, chop garlic and other ingredients into a smooth paste. Sprinkle with salt and set aside for a few hours. Add olive oil and mix. <|endoftext|>

Burgers

In a medium bowl, combine turkey, onion, jalapeño, salsa, garlic, oregano, and salt. Evenly divide the mixture into four patties, about $4, and grill them at medium heat until cooked through and the internal meat thermometer registers 160°F to 165°F and the meat no longer appears pink. To serve, place the burgers on sliced bun bottoms

Agriculture is how cities and nations were founded.

Honey sweet and sour meatballs

Courtesy of the American Beekeeping Federation https://www.abfnet.org

Ingredients:

1 ½ lbs of ground beef

1 ½ teaspoons season salt

½ cup milk

½ teaspoon pepper

½ cup butter

½ cup honey

¼ cup vinegar.

1 medium onion, cut into

1-inch sections

2 tablespoons soy sauce

1 8 oz can pineapple with juice

¼ teaspoon teaspoon cayenne pepper or to taste

2 tablespoons cornstarch

2 ounces water

Directions:

Make meatballs from ground beef, and add some soy sauce and cayenne for color. Pepper with freshly ground black pepper. Mix thoroughly. Form meat into balls with hands and cook them in hot cooking oil. As they are cooking, add some juice from a can of pineapple to the pan, along with some water and onion juice from white onion. Cook this sauce for a few minutes down low. Combine cornstarch and water to make a paste. Add to the pan to thicken as it reduces and cooks down slightly shiny. Dredge the meatballs in the sticky sweet/sour sauce

Ravioli with an Italian meat sauce

Self-esteem through others

(www.Ilovepasta.com) Serves 4-6

Ingredients:

A cup pound pasta, uncooked

Try It & Get 8 grams.

Make broth with bones.

Parsley

Six large tomatoes, peeled, seeded and diced

½-1 teaspoon salt

1/2 teaspoon dried oregano.

½ teaspoon dried basil

½ teaspoon sugar

1 Tablespoon red wine

Directions:

Prepare the pasta according to the package directions; as soon as it's ready, blend together the onion, meat, and garlic; then stir the mole into the spaghetti. Simmer for about 20 minutes, or up to 20 minutes if you add more mole ingredients. When the pasta is cooked, drain it. Put a couple of spoonfuls of mole into

All you need for a great weeknight meal

Duty to our civilization

(www.nysmaple.com)

Ingredients:

½ cup granulated processed

Two shallots, peeled and sliced

One ounce fresh thyme

½ cup water

1 tablespoon kosher salt.

1/2 teaspoon pepper

2 pounds

Directions:

Combine maple syrup, shallots, thyme, water and salt, then cook and boil until sugar is dissolved; cool. Skim fat from broth; serve.

Whipped Grilled Steak stuffed with Pumpkin Puree

Serves 4

Ingredients:

19 Pork rib eyes

4 medium potatoes chopped

6 ounces of chopped pumpkin meat.

1 tablespoon butter

¼ cup milk

Salt and pepper, to taste

Directions:

Place cooked potatoes in soup and add pumpkin. Continue to cook until very tender. Drain and mash well, adding a little butter and milk to thicken. Lightly season and sauté steaks over hot coals. Grill steaks for 4 minutes. Cover grill and cook for 3 to 4 minutes for medium rare. Season with salt and serve with the mashed pumpkin. <|endoftext|>

Broiled steak with spicy mustard and apple chutney

funding from NHLBI, NIH/HHS

Ingredients: Chutney

A Granny Smith apple, rinsed, peeled, cored, and diced (about 1 cup)

2 medium shallots

⅛ Tablespoon garlic

½ cup canned no-salt-added diced tomatoes

2 tablespoons golden seedless raisins (about ½ cup)

As much as ¼ cup apple cider vinegar

Two spoonfuls of pure maple syrup.

Steak

These are 4

¼ teaspoon salt

1/4 teaspoon ground pepper

1 teaspoon olive oil

Mustard Dressing

2 tablespoons Dijon mustard

2 tablespoons cornstarch

Directions: Chutney

Assemble all the ingredients in a saucepan. Bring the mixture to a rolling boil and boil for 20 minutes or until the apples are cooked well and soft. Hold the mixture warm, or cool it and store it.

Steak

Heat up what kind of grill pan or oven broiler? Prep some meat that you like making it seasoned? Then, enjoy the great taste of steak! MMMMGood!

Mustard Dressing

Combine six cups of beef broth with a dash of mustard and cornstarch; bring the mixture to a boil on medium heat, while stirring it constantly. Lower the heat, and simmer until the beef broth is well blended and the mixture thickens, usually just a couple minutes. Serve each steak with ¼ cup of ch

Braised Corned Beef with Maple

Courtesy of the Massachusetts Maple Producers Association

(www.massmaple.org)

Ingredients:

4 pounds premium corned beef, dry-cured

Apple

¼ cup Spirits

Directions:

Place dried sliced brisket in roasting pan and bake uncovered in the oven at 325°F for thirty minutes. Reduce the heat to 275F and cover. Baking Can 1 hour. Uncover, discard all but ½ cup Liquid, adding in maple syrup and bourbon (if using). Continue baking and basting frequently for an additional

Roast Pork Loin with Apples

I wish the National Honey Board was always around

(www.honey.com)

Ingredients:

1½ pounds pork loin

1 tablespoon of olive oil

3 teaspoons of ground black pepper

1/2 spoon ground ginger

½ teaspoon nutmeg

½ teaspoon cinnamon

Enjoy 1/2 of dry white wine

1 Tablespoon lemon juice

¼ cup honey

Cut 2 big apples into wedges

Directions:

Mix the pork loin with extra-virgin olive oil, cracked black pepper, half of chopped ginger, star anise, nutmeg, and cinnamon. Combine remaining half of spices with wine, lemon juice, and honey; stir in apple slices. Bake at 350

Put pork into a shallow baking pan. Pop it into the oven until the pork reaches an internal temperature of about 155 degrees. Parchment parchment paper and/or foil around the pan to catch and transfer melting juices as it bakes. To pull it off the heat

Simmer the apple mix until it's tender and add any juices from the pork and any other ingredients. Simmer another several minutes.

Pork loin and sa...

A slice of pork (called a 'mignon') with fresh applesauce (FRENCH APPLESAUCE)

Courtesy of the NHLBI, part of the NIHR and the Department of Health and Human Services.

Ingredients:

50 pounds 6 of tomatoes 6

¼ teaspoon salt

Peppercorn

½ cup water

2 medium, rinsed, but not cored, Apples, Golden Delicious or Rome

2 tablespoons dried cranberries

2.5 tbsp. walnuts, broken into large pieces

½ teaspoon cinnamon

Cooking spray

Directions:

Turn up the oven's broiler. Place the pan in the oven and turn the oven on to high heat.

To replicate commercial recipes, cut each pork tenderloin in half and cut each half into eight slices about one and a half inches thick. Place the pork slices on a broiler pan covered with aluminum foil. Sprinkle with salt and pepper, and let the oven heat.

As he watched, the zenne cooked in a medium heat. "Cut the apples in wedges or slices ¼ inch - wide," he noted. Why I love section writing: On your own, expand on

Preheat oven to 400°F. Place apples and raisins in a 9x5-inch baking dish. Add walnuts and cinnamon to the apple mixture and mix well. Add pork to the apple mixture and coat well

Roast pork tenderloins for 5-10 minutes per side (for a minimum internal temperature of 160°F) and then serve. Serve each slice of pork with ¼ of apple sauce and 3 forbidden bread sticks.

Note: Simplify the Sauce or serve over whole-wheat pancakes.

Apples, the best guilt-free snack

• Foods contain zero fats, cholesterol, or sodium.

One medium apple has only about 80 calories.

• apples

[Multiply] Baked Pork Chops with Apple Cranberry Sauce

your health

Ingredients: Pork Chops

4 Boneless Pork Chops (about three ounces each)

Black is for good luck and represents visibility and wealth

½ teaspoon

Mix ½ tablespoon olive oil in some water.

Sauce

¼ cup chicken broth

about 1/2 cup peeled and grated apple <|endoftext|>

(Use a grater to make thin layers of and apple)

For cinnamon, one teaspoon of ground cinnamon

1 bay leaf

½ more cup dried cranberries

½ cup 200ml 100% orange juice

Directions: Pork Chops

Cube chop a loaf of baguette and place in the oven to toast. Season pork loins with pepper and sprinkle cinnamon. Heat a large sauté pan over medium- high heat, and coat the pan with olive oil. Add pork loins, and brown on both sides, about 2 to 3 minutes on each side (use a spatula to even out the cooking). Move to a large baking pan. Bake to a golden brown and within

Sauce

Because some broth needs to be saved in the fridge to use later, the only other thing to do is to add it to chicken broth to make a delicious dish. This way, when you have leftover broth, you can make some cold chicken soup.

Notes: An amazing fruit sauce to serve over Your pork chops. Try serving with brown rice and broccoli.

Pork chumps

Courtesy of the NY State Maple Producers Association.

(www.nysmaple.com)

Ingredients:

1½ cups pure maple syrup

35 ml of distilled water

¼ cup horseradish

1 teaspoon ancho chile powder

4-8 pork chops

Directions:

Preheat the oven to 400 degrees Fahrenheit. Mix the maple syrup with the white wine, vinegar, dried horseradish, and chili powder well. Bake the bell peppers whole in the oven for about an hour. Serve a sprinkling of freshly grated horseradish, or mixed horseradish with chilies.

Error creating thumbnail: Could not find URL at Honey Chinese BBQ Pork

The benefits of honey are so happening and widespread. The journal "Benefits of honey" is is. n the first place on the list of health benefits and benefits of honey is the number

(www.benefits-of-honey.com)

Ingredients:

Two pounds of pork

2 cloves of garlic, blended and ground

¼ teaspoon five spices powder

Add 1⁄2 tablespoon soy sauce

½ teaspoon pepper

1 teaspoon salt

Add 1/4 cup margarine or vegetable oil to *The best way to look good in a swimsuit

4-5 tablespoons of honey (a rose honey variety works well)

Directions:

Chop the lean pork tenderly and marinate it in the fridge for about 5 hours. Season it with spices, soy sauce, salt, pepper and sugar. Hang the pieces of fried pork up to dry. As soon as they start to dry, you have to grill the pork slices until both sides are golden, and brush them with margarine. Add honey from time to time and serve hot. If you decide to freeze them, carry out the procedure, but don't flip them over. This will enable you to grill their sides before serving.

Tenderloin stuffed with marinated pork, skipped salt

Choose the input that provides the best customer experience.

(www.americangrassfed.org) Serves 6-8

Ingredients: Fresh Tomato Sauce

1¾ pouns Roma tomatoes (see Note)

1 teaspoon olive oil

¼ cup

Add one clove of minced garlic, maybe two or three, some salt.

½ cup tomato paste

Safely drink 2 cans of chicken or vegetable stock (or more as needed)

2 Tablespoons fresh basil, chopped<|endoftext|>

Seasoning: salt and freshly ground black pepper to taste

Pork

How do you calculate inches?

1 (4 oz.) log of fres unsalted goat cheese

3 cloves of garlic, minced

2 tablespoons asparagus

½ teaspoon salt

½⁄2 tablespoon freshly ground pepper

1 tablespoon olive oil

Iced mint tea

Salt, pepper, and your choice of other spices

Begin with directions.

Don't peel and chop your tomatoes yet. Start them in the giant sauté pan that you heat up at the stove. The fat from the olive oil is the best way to flavor the sauce and help it thicken up. The red color comes from grapeseed oil, so dunk tomatoes in this to keep them from being too bland (not like pickled grapes or Vidalia onions). This project with the sauce is to add things like basil, salt and pepper,

Pork

If the tomato sauce bakes along time in the oven, the pork loin marinates in goat cheese, olive oil, rosemary, and garlic paste. The smoky-tasting pork loin gets kicked up with a simple sprinkle of salt and pepper. To carve and serve, the logs of bacon are simmering at 400°F. While biting the edge of that ceramic baking dish, the loins of pork are folded together, sliced, and sprinkled with rosemary. The whole dish of pork surround by the trail of tomato sauce is set in a low oven. The recipe says 15 minutes per side. Given cooking times for roasting temperatures for pork, the pork loins must be turned until enough heat is applied to the crust, enough time is allowed for heat to penetrate to the

Note: If you can't find ripe gourmet tomatoes, you can improve the flavor by roasting the tomatoes today. Cut the tomatoes in half lengthwise, seed them, and place them cut - side up on a baking sheet. Roast in a 325°F oven for about

Say you want to reduce the strong tomato flavor often found in canned tomatoes. Allow the tomatoes to simmer in a covered pan on the stove for about 20 minutes and watch carefully so that no burns occurs. Don't overcook, though, or the tomato paste will pinche

Maple Baked Ham

Guest Access Area: Grassy area, Dart Boards, Play equipment

(www.shaverhillfarm.com)

Ingredients:

Heat/simmer/melt butter in a nonstick skillet over medium heat while whisking. When the butter is almost done, add

2/3 cups lemon juice

¾ c cup pure maple syrup

It seems that there are 6-8 slices of ham.

Directions:

Mix mustard seeds and lemon juice, and stir until smooth. Add a little maple syrup, then pour over sliced ham in a pan that will fit the ham in one layer, and bake for 50 minutes, basting every 10 minutes.

Baked Fresh Tomato, Ham, and Swiss Rolls Perfect natural dietary suggestions

The Florida Tomato Growers Association

(www.floridatomatoes.org) Serves 4

Ingredients:

2 dozen large fresh tomatoes

6-ounces of thinly sliced ham

Six 1½ cup ounces shredded Swiss cheese

3 tablespoons creamy mustard

How can you start working out?

4 large, hard round (Kaiser) rolls, halved

Directions:

Use large chunks of sweet, juicy tomatoes, and large pieces of ham and cheese as serving pieces. Remove the middle part of each of the rolls, leaving ½inch thick sheet.

Foie Gras

Ingredients: Roast Duck

1. Duck, washed and dried

6 cupes bread crumbs

6 ounces butter

2 onions, chopped

1 teaspoon sage

1 teaspoon pepper

1 teaspoon salt

Heat, salt, limited amounts of butter, and flour for basting

Currant Jelly Sauce

3 tablespoons butter

1 onion

1 tablespoon flour

1 bay leaf

1 sprig celery

One pint of poultry stock

2 tablespoons vinegar

½ cup crusant jelly

Salt and pepper to taste

Directions: Roast Duck

On its original form, this Duck was cleaned thoroughly and the surface was wiped dry. Cut the neck close to the back. Next, blend butter, ingredients like onions, sage, garlic, pepper, and salt, and stuff it into the bird. Lightly baste the bird with salt, initially, as well as salty water, and then stop basting if you'd like. Safe baking time is 25 to 30 minutes depending on the age of the bird-around 1 hour is the safe baking time for the Rite brand. Baste the bird with butter, salt and water and you probably will add spices if you want. Young ducks should be baked for 30 to 35 minutes and the full grown ones for about 40 minutes. Sometimes

Currant Jelly Sauce

In the summer rolling boil the butter and onion until the onion begins to turn yellow. As the onions is coloring, add the flour. Stir over heat until starting to brown. Add the stock and vinegar, and simmer 20 minutes. Remove the pan from the stove and skim off all the fat. Add the jelly, being careful to melt it completely.

HEALTH BENEFIT OF BERRIES</

The pigment makeup that gives berries their vibrant colors also make them an excellent for your health.

Berries such as blueberries, raspberries and strawberries contain many phytonutrients, which are believed to promote good health. For this reason, they are considered as convenient and great sources of the boosting substances.

Shepherd's Pie

Courtesy of Hood River Garlic Farm

(www.hoodrivergarlic.com) Serves 4

Ingredients: Pie

1½ pounds of organic ground baby back ribs

1 medium onion

3 chopped carrots

1 teaspoon of sliced garlic

1 tablespoon rosemary

¼ cup chicken or beef stock.

Approximately<|endoftext|>

1 tablespoon flour

Salt and pepper, to taste

Crust

2 quarts water

7 medium potatoes, chopped

3 tablespoons butter

3 tablespoons garlic

½ cup whole milk.

Salt and pepper to taste

Directions: Pie

Heat pre-heat the oven to 450°F. Brown the ground beef, drain off fat and simmer it in the skillet until the beef is cooked but not over done. Add the onions, carrots, garlic and rosemary. Break them up and add chicken or beef stock. Simmer and let the stock dries. Add the green pepper. Let all the stock evaporate and combine the flour with the meat mixture. Make sure to drain off excess liquid. Pour the mixture in a pie dish and let it cool while you make the crust mixture.

Crust

I was wondering if I could sneak some of Daddy's fries into today's dinner because I don't want to be bothered with preparing mashed potatoes. Can you help me please? And do you think I should put on some of my sunscreen because I'm going out fishing today?

Perfect Honey Pizza

Processed honey is found to be the winner in its health benefits. The top ranked website claims - 'The number one ranked website on the health benefits of hone- y .'

(www.benefits-of-honey.com)

Ingredients:

1-2 Tablespoons honey, try Fireweed or Tawari varieties.

5 slices of soft white bread

3 tomatoes

Waffle: Cut ham into 1- × 1-inch squares

10 Tablespoons of shredded mozzarella cheese

Directions:

Spread Tuami Chutney on bread slices. Lay on the tomatoes followed by ham pieces on top. Then spread on the cheese and finish placing in the oven at 285°F. <|endoftext|>

Hot Hot Freezer Meatballs

Courtesy of the Garlic seed Foundation These red arrows are used because, well, they are rare, and we're sure our targeting keyword picks don

(www.garlicseedfoundation.info)

Ingredients:

1 egg

1/2 head large garlic

Love Vodka by Chanel No 5

¼ cup or less hot sauce (or less "heat")

1 pound ground beef

¾ cup quick cooking oatmeal <|endoftext|>

½ cup Parmesan cheese

1 teaspoon coarse ground black pepper

½ teaspoon salt (optional) **Note: Here, we've chopped up a sentence. Typically a paraphrase would be a

Use 1½ teaspoons Italian

½ teaspoon each chopped fresh basil and oregano

Directions:

Pre-heat the oven to 450˚F. Saute garlic and onion in a drippings pan, until brown. Cool and blend in a food processor with meat, then add remaining ingredients. Shapes meatballs, wrap the balls in cling film, then twist or freeze.

These make a versatile and quick meal when paired with quick stir-fries and pasta or in pasta or stir-fry sauces. The dish is very flexible and can be paired with a number of different sauces.

A large number of you may be vegetarian, more so than any other type of "food". A healthy vegetable is considered a "meal". So many of you may have discovered vegetarian entrees, you may have found vegan meals. If so, another option may be if you could include a protein

A palatable food that is easily digestible is needed to satisfy all people eight hours per day, seven days per week. The issue of meat is used as a political wedge to classify people into we or they self-identified groups, supporting "our" group by using it to promote "their" group. People are beginning to question the modus operandi of large meat organizations. They will never give up until the lyrics of the Meat Puppets become an accepted myth. People are choosing to rinse their under

Vegetarian entrees certainly shouldn't be tasteless. In fact, the smart use of spices, herbs, and vegetable ingredients in healthy recipes like Chili, Tomatoes with Roasted Red Peppers, and Fresh Basil (this page), Pasta with Tomatoes, Roasted Red Peppers, and Fresh Basil (this page), and Mexibean Cheese Lasagna (this page) will tempt your appetite and your taste buds so completely that you will forget that these are meat-free dishes. In this section, you can find the unpacking of beneficial gluten-free, vegan meat alternatives perfect for every traditional, beautifully

Cabbage and Pumpkin Stir-Fry

Serves 4

Ingredients:

2 teaspoons oil

An onion, diced

1 minced garlic clove

1 Jumbag of ginger root

about two medium sized cups (200g) of pumpkin meat.

2 large green onions, chopped

This salad is crunchy and packed with fiber

1 tablespoon lime juice, cornstarch, and water

1 teaspoon sesame oil

One tablespoon of sesame seeds

Pepper, to taste

Directions:

In a pan, heat the grapeseed oil over medium-high heat. Add onions, garlic, ginger, and pumpkin, and cook until the onions are translucent. Add green onions, cabbage, and water. Stir-fry for 10 minutes or until pumpkin is soft. Add soy sauce (or ketchup), and stir well. Now add cornstarch and water, mixing well so that vegetables do not stick. Drizzle with

Celery and Apple Steam Fry with honey-Mustard Sauce

Ingredients:

1 cup water

Four cups cubed celery, ½-inch thick slices

Fresh red berries are good for you.

1 tbsp

1 tablespoon honey

1 teaspoon cornstarch

¼ teaspoon black pepper

¼ cup chopped toasted walnuts (optional)

Directions:

In a large skillet, bring 10 cups of water to boil and add celery and apples; cook and stir until crisp-tender, about 8 minutes, adding more water if necessary. Cook the celery and onions as described above. Once the onions are cooked, combine the ingredients in a blender and blend until smooth. Sprinkle on the walnuts, if desired. Serve over rice.

Fruity Curried Lentils

Ingredients:

2 cups of uncooked lentils

2 quarts water

2 apples par-sealed, cored and chopped.

Carrots, half of ¼ cup golden raisins

Two-thirds of a cup

Cook the curry one tsp. at a time

½ teaspoon salt

Directions:

Combine Lentils with water and stir Together. Bring to a boil, reduce heat, and simmer 20 minutes, stirring often. Stir in Apples and Raisins, placing donuts in large container (liked out) and covering. Chill until ready to serve.

Roasted garlic and a healthy atmosphere. <|endoftext|>

Courtesy of Hood River Garlic Farm

(www.hoodrivergarlic.com)

Ingredients:

1 pound (4.5 oz) carrots, peeled

1 pound of carrots, cleaned

1 large sweet potato without the skin

1 tub of unsweetened coconut milk (about 1 cup)

1 bulb of garlic, peeled

5 Tablespoons of Extra-Virgin Olive Oil.

1teaspoon salt

½ teaspoon crushed black peppercorns

2 tablespoons chopped parsley

Directions:

Start the oven to 425°F and turn it on. Cut the carrots, parsnips, sweet potato, and squash into 1- to 1¼ inch cubes. Grate the garlic. Put the vegetables into a large bowl, drizzle with olive oil and sprinkle them with salt, pepper, and parsley; toss well. Transfer the vegetables onto two sheet pans. After the first 15 minutes, mix the vegetables so that they don't

Stripe: A marbled purple to mocha colored stripe would look great on the body of the matt.

vegetables with spicy honey peanut sauce

Be courteous

(www.honey.com)

Ingredients:

½ cup honey

What's a ¼ cup worth?

30.4gms soy sauce or 1 tablespoon

I like it hot, I like it hot.

⅛ teaspoon crushed red pepper flakes

A cup of broccoli has 4 cups

4 cups of sliced carrots 4 carrots

4 tablespoons snow peas

4 cups cooked white rice

Directions:

Mix honey, peanut butter, soy sauce, cilantro, and red peppers in a small bowl. Let it sit for 10 minutes while you steam veggies. Dress the veggies with the peanut sauce and eat when ready.

Try our Spicy Grilled Tofu

Be nice when you lead.

(www.honey.com)

Ingredients:

8 slices of 14.2 oz. package Extra firm tofu

One ½ cup of fresh lime juice

cup honey

1 4 cup soy sauce

2 teaspoons chili paste with garlic

2 cloves garlic, minced

¼ teaspoon ground pepper

Directions:

Place tofu slices on several layers of paper towels; cover with additional paper towels. Let stand 20 minutes, pressing down occasionally with your hands to squeeze out water. Arrange tofu in single layer in 13- × 9-inch glass baking dish. Whisk together lime juice, honey, soy sauce, chili paste, garlic, and pepper in small bowl. Pour over tofu, coating each slice. Cover tightly with plastic wrap and chill 4 hours or overnight. Spray grill rack or pan with non-stick cooking spray. Heat grill or grill pan to medium heat. Remove tofu slices from baking dish, reserving marinade. Grill tofu slices 3 to 4 minutes on each side or until browned and crisp on the outside. Return tofu to baking dish and toss with reserved marinade. Serve immediately.

Aaaaoooonne Pumpin Tomnoshtt

Ingredients:

3½ pounds pumpkin

1 onion, chopped A: I'm pretty positive the intent of both posts was to inspire readers to become better at

Make broth of tomatoes

1 tablespoon margarine

Use 1 tablespoon of cooking oil

1/4 cup is made out of 1 shallot

2 teaspoons salt

Toast

Directions:

Wash and pare the pumpkin and cut into 2-inch square pieces. Put the pumpkin into a frying pan, and fry the chopped onions until brown. Add the pumpkin, salt, and pepper, and then cook for five minutes. Cover the pumpkin with the tomatoes, and stew gently until it is soft. Mix the tomato into the pumpkin and add enough lemon juice to thicken the tomato. Season with more salt and pepper if needed. Pour over the pumpkin and garnish with

Pumpkin Timbale

Ingredients:

STAP ($4.75)

1 tablespoon grapeseed oil

2 to 3 ounces ricotta cheese

1 teaspoon vanilla extract

2 Egg Pockets are large

Large pinch meringue

2 eggs

Salt and pepper to taste

Directions:

What we are going to do today is to take a basic stove top technique and make it a euristic method for if someone shouts at you.

Pumpkin and Ginger Coconut Sauce

Serves 4

Ingredients:

Pumpkin size just under one pound cut into pieces

1 tablespoon grapeseed oil

8 scallions, sliced

1 blade of fresh ginger, crushed

1 crushed and seeded jalapeño

1/2 (14.5 oz.) can unsweetened regular coconut milk

1 teaspoon curry paste.

2 tablespoons of freshly minced cilantro

Salt and pepper, to suit your taste.

Directions:

Heat the oil in a large pan. Add the chunks of pumpkin and sauté until slightly brown. Add scallions, ginger, jalapeño, coconut milk, curry paste, cilantro, and bring to a boil over medium heat. Reduce heat, and cook until the pumpkin is tender, about 15-20 minutes. Add a little water, if the sauce becomes too thick. Add some salt

It's good **lunch** pot-roast over rice.

Chickpea Veg Pak

Serves 6

Ingredients:

1 cup onion, chopped

Chop or grate 1½ cups fresh ginger

Go for 1 tablespoon

Olive oil ½ teaspoon less?

1 cup drained chickpeas (referring to 19 oz. can of chickpeas)

14 cups

1 cup of fresh spinach. No stems.

½ cup water

¼ teaspoon

Directions:

This heart-healthy meal can be made easily with a food processor. Mash up the onion mixture and add the curry; then add the chickpeas and tomato along with spinach leaves. Mix well, continue cooking while stirring until the spinach wilts. Add water, salt and brown rice or any other grain of your choice, and either add whatever you would normally add

If you can't afford a food processor, chop onions and ginger finely. A blender or the stick blender found in most kitchens can also be used to fine chop.

Grilled tofu salad

Protecting honey

(www.honey.com)

Ingredients: Chipotle Marinade

1/2 cup vegetable broth

Use only enough white: garlic to give flavor to a dish

cup honey

1/2 cup of tamari soy sauce

Skillet, Onion, Cabbage

Izmalda ocho espeso

1 ¼ teaspoons granulated onion powder

1 tablespoon of Dijon mustard

1 teaspoon finely chopped cilantro

Grilled Tofu Kabobs

2 (14 oz.)

2 avocados and some Chipotle marinade

3 medium zucchini

1-inch circles

Cut into 1-inch chunks

1 medium red onion, chopped

1-inch wedges

12 cherry tomatoes

1 pineapple and water cup

Directions: Marinade

Combine melted butter, garlic paste, chipotle in adobo, soy, and honey. Mix well. Add spices, and adobo.

Kabobs

Slice each block of tofu in half horizontally. Then slice the block of tofu in half vertically and horizontally. Soak bamboo skewers then thread tofu, veggies, and pineapples together. Place over low coals and cover the grill. Cook the kabobs for 20 to 30 minutes, or until done. While heating chop ingredients and drain. Add ingredients to large glass baking dish. With oven mitts, remove slide sheet and pour salad dressing on top of tofu salad. Stir ingredients to mix and serve.

GRADES OF HONEY

Farmstands usually offer honey in a variety of different flavors, that can vary in certain amounts. Personalized Paraphrases

Grade 12 honey can be extracted that scores: **a minimum of 90 out of 100 points** on the grading

Grade B honey must receive at least 80 points.

Standard honey scores at least 70 out of 100 points. Any honey that receives less than 70 points goes into **Grade "C" honey**.

Easter Egg Peppers With Eggplant, Tomatoes and Sesame Rice And with Pineapple, Sesame Rice, and Sweet

Courtesy of www.ILoveEggplant.com

Ingredients: Skewers

1 an inch wedges of Japanese eggplant

1-inch wedges

Cut up bell pepper

With 1-inch by 1-inch sections

8 cherry tomatoes per serving

1-inch by

1-inch sections

8 button mushrooms

Mae Hawthorne Hamentz Sweet Chili Sauce, for dipping

Directions: Skewers

Stick, i.e. Mom Thats talking about a concept named skewers, alternating with other vegetables.

Rice

Remove the rice from the stockpot, wash it and get ready to cook it. Place all rice preparation ingredients in a saucepot. Bring stockpot to a boil, covered. Bun the preparation and serve the rice and kabobs together.

NOTE: If you are using wooden skewers, one way to prevent them from burning on the grill is to soak them overnight in water. This can help keep the skewers from catching on fire!

Grain Cayenne

Serves 4

Ingredients: Dip

1 cup chopped pineapples.

1/4 cup apple juice

¼ cup plain non-fat yogurt

Fruit

2 bananas

one teaspoon of orange juice

38 fruit slices, each cut an inch thick.

1 cup purple, seedless grapes

Eat 3 strawberries today.

cup green melon balls

cup blackberries

Directions: Dip

Your friends won't believe this has pineapple and apple juice in it: you MUST introduce it to them!

Fruit

You make the dip by placing oranges, kiwi slices, bananas, kiwi quarters, grape pieces, strawberry sections, melon balls, and blackberries together in a small bowl. Drizzle orange juice over the fruit, and mash a little for a creamier texture. Serve over hum

See more tips for storing fruits and veggies.

• Buy and snip open good berries. Then place overripe or moldy ones in a different container. Finally, you can remove the good berries and place proper in a secure container of your choosing.

• Rinse berries

• Do not let apple and pear slices sit in the sun; they must be stored in a refrigerator set at 32°F - 40°F.

• Berries can be stored in an airtight container that will keep them in good condition. Contrary to the advice of some written in the Dr. Oz Show article, berries should be stored with sugar in order to preserve the healthiest taste for longer periods.

• Legumes and berries can be preserved into a variety of jellies, jams, salsas, and chutneys.

Stuffed Ferme-Milieux Peppers

Respect the honey

(www.honey.com)

Ingredients:

1 - tablespoon vegetable or olive oil

¾ cup cooked long grain rice

2 basil, fresh, julienned

¼ cup finely chopped fresh parsley

¼ teaspoon cinnamon.

¼ teaspoons black pepper or cayenne pepper

¼ teaspoon salt

Add 1 cup vegetable broth to a pot or microwaveable container. Set the ingredients aside to cool.

2 medium green bell peppers, cut lengthwise in half and seeded

1 (28 oz.) can crushed tomatoes in puree

¼ cup honey

½ teaspoon crushed red pepper flakes

1¼ cups garbanzo beans, drained

½ cup dried currants or raisins

Directions:

While the Chicken Tenders sizzle in the pan, his smart Cookie mashes up some of his lettuce mix in their juices so they have lots of healthy added veggies. He flutters his Garnish Mind over the Chicken Tenders and the peaches to make sure every morsel is coated in the delicious sauce. The last morsel is a dessert for us because we always love it when he does this.

A Garlic Roasted Garlic Grilled Cheese Sandwich

Courtesy

(www.torontogarlicfestival.ca) Serves 1

Ingredients:

1 Tablespoon Roasted Garlic Puree (see recipe on this page)

2 slices of whole wheat or multi grain bread

these two slices of cheese

30 milliliters of a low-fat substitute butter

Directions:

Start out by spreading a thin layer of roasted garlic on only one side of one slice of bread. Put the cheese in the middle and spread butter on the outside of the sandwich. Turn the sandwich for color side down in a pan over medium heat. When one side has turned golden brown, turn it over and prepare to serve. The sandwich is cut in half and garnished with sliced pickled garlic scapes.

Gail tried to make an Salem-Dale jelly from the garlic scapes growing in their front yard. She had particularly high hopes for it, considering how pretty they were.

Honey of a chili

Hesitation to show kindness

(www.honey.com)

Ingredients:

1 (15 oz.) package (cubed) firm tofu

1 teaspoon vegetable oil

1 large chopped onion

1 cup of chopped green bell pepper

Garlic Raw harissa

1 tablespoon chili powder

1 Teaspoon ground Cardamom

1 teaspoon salt

Ommeges – half an teaspoon oregano flakes

½ teaspoon crushed red pepper flakes

Only (28 oz.) can diced tomatoes

1 (15oz.) can red kidney beans, undrained

1 (8 oz.) can tomato sauce

¼ cup honey

2 tablespoons red wine vinegar

Directions:

Using a cheese grater, cut tofu and freeze twelve hours or up to two days. Thaw tofu and drain well by pressing with a rack or cheesecloth over a saucepan. Put paper towels in a strainer and pour on tofu. Put tofu in a saucepan with a bit of cold water and let it stand in low heat, fifteen to thirty minutes or until water gets hot and starts to boil so that tofu puffs up a bit. Then cut up the other hits (tofu and baking soda) like in this video:

A quick Spinach Casserole

Serves 8

Ingredients:

3 packages

2 cups non-fat cottage cheese

1 large banana

¼ cup flour

½ teaspoon salt

Should I add chicken liver paté or some other spread?

Directions:

Simply mix all ingredients together. Pour into a low-temperature slow-cooker and cook on low. Cook for 4 hours.

Spicy Apple-Filled Squash

Ingredients:

1 acorn squash (1 lb.)

1 apple

Two teaspoons reduced fat margarine melted

2 tsp brown sugar

⅛ teaspoon cinnamon

⅛ teaspoon nutmeg

Dash ground cloves

Directions:

Heat the oven to 350 F. Grease a 1-quart baking dish; place squash in dish, cut sides up and cover; bake for 30 minutes. Meanwhile, combine apple, butter with brown sugar, cinnamon, nutmeg, and cloves in medium bowl; discard crusts from squash halves; spoon apple mixture onto squash; cover and bake 30 minutes longer or until squash and apple are tender

Microwave version: Follow salad version recipe as stated, except substitute coconut milk + coconut powder for fat-free yogurt + nonfat Greek yogurt. Add almond sprinkles for the topping and the lid for the microwave as authorities advise using them.

The Mexibean Cheese Lasagna

Serves 6

Ingredients:

2 tablespoons olive oil

1½ teaspoons chopped onion

3 cloves of garlic

1 green pepper, coarsely chopped

1/2 teaspoon of ground red pepper

one teaspoon ground cumin

2 tablespoons chili powder.

½ teaspoon cayenne powder

One cup frozen corn kernels

1 teaspoon tomato paste ** Original: 1 (15 oz.) can red kidney beans, rinsed and drained Paraphrase: (40 mins.)

1 can (15 oz. serving size) black beans; rinse; drain

Tomato sauce lower in sodium

1 (4 oz.) can diced green chilies, drained

Non-stick cooking spray

6 corn tortillas

One cup fat-free ricotta cheese

One and a half Tbsp. of low-fat cheddar cheese, shredded

Directions:

In large skillet, heat some oil over medium heat. In an aside, cook the onion, garlic, and peppers. Add the spices and saute the spices for an additional minute to flavor the onions. Whisk the cooked corn, beans, tomato sauce, and diced green chilies into the onions and veggie mixture. Spread half of the corn mixture across the tortillas, and ricotta and cheddar cheese on top. Repeat, using up all the ingredients. Cook, uncovered at about 350°F for about 45 minutes, until cooked all the way through and casserole has melted. Serve immediately.

Macaroni and Cheese

Ingredients:

4 cups macaroni

14% fat, 2 medium eggs and 1/2 cup thinly sliced red onion

2-4 tablespoons butter

1 tablespoon flour

1 cup milk

2 cups cream

Salt and black pepper

Directions:

1- Break macaroni into pieces in the large pan with rapidly boiling salted water. 2- Boil macaroni until it can stick to a fork. 3- Remove from heat, drain, then have grated cheese about ½ hour before serving. 4- make a heaping tablespoon of butter in a separate pan. Turn on low heat slowly. Affect stirring constantly. Add small amounts of flour and stir until it is smooth and thick. Stir in unsweetened cream and butter in quick succession. Stir

Pasta Primavera

Ingredients:

1 cup broccoli florets

1 cup of sliced carrots

1 cup sliced zucchini

1 cup of macaroni or rotini pasta

Sauce

1 tablespoon margarine

1 tablespoon flour

1 cup of skim milk cooked

½ tsp basil TC: Try Different Athletes (Paraphrase is a portion of a paraphrase, but the whole sentence is

⅛ teaspoon of black pepper

2.5 tablespoons Parmesan cheese

Directions:

Steam vegetables until crisp-tender, and cook macaroni according to package directions.

Sauce

The original recipe calls for melting the margarine in a small pot. After the margarine is melted, the cook should slowly add milk to the pot until it is thick. An important point is to not to add cheese at this time. The cook could slowly stir in the cheese to serve the sauce over the hot starch covered vegetables.

back to CookPaste

Serves 6

Ingredients:

As the bulb of a fresh garlic

6 cups vegetables (eg., 1 cup each of cubed eggplant, zucchini, and yellow squash, 2 cups elm beans, 2 cups tomatoes,

1/4 cup to 1/2 cup balsamic vinegar

2 tablespoons

¼ tsp dried oregano

½ teaspoon fresh chopped pepper

3 cups (about 3 medium) chopped tomatoes

10 oz.-12 oz. large bow tie pasta

2 tablespoons fresh parsley.

¼ –cup[1] cup freshly grated Parmesan cheese

Directions:

Two parts eggplant stir into one well-seasoned (garlic, oregano and salt). Set aside. Mix in a bowl. Add vinegar, extra wine of olives, salt and lightly-dried peppers. Let sit for an hour. Grill a chopped vine of tomatoes and garlic. Cook pasta in boiling water according to directions. Split eggplant sheets in half like toilet paper and stack half on top of cooked pasta. Cover with equal amounts of unison tomato-garlic mixture and parsley of saltiness. Garnish with Parmesan cheese. Serve immediately.

Thai Noodles & Snow Peas

Honey has been proven to clean your body and ward off bacteria.

(www.honey.com)

Ingredients:

Tofu cut into ½-inch pieces

1 (9 oz.) package fresh Asian noodles

Green peas, peeled, cut diagonally and 8 ounces.

A quarter cup of chopped cilantro

Marinade

1/3 cup rice vinegar

¼ cup honey

2 tablespoons.

2 tablespoons soya sauce.

2 tablespoons canola oil. Steps: • Get canola oil and heat • Mix all ingredients • Wait 20 minutes

1 tablepoon of sesame oil

The initial reduced cost of modern fruits and vegetables

1/2 tsp crushed red pepper

¼ teaspoon ground ginger

Directions:

In medium bowl, combine marinade ingredients. Add tofu; marinate 30 minutes Whirl noodles and snow peas in 3 quarts boiling water one to two minutes. Rinse with cold water. Drain. Place in a large bowl; add tofu and marinade. Stir to coat soy tofu. Top with green onions and cilantro.<|endoftext|>

Tomatoes, Roasted red peppers, and Fresh basil Use these steps to paraphrase the next 12 lines in CoffeeScript. It is good to review both

The work of the Central New York Tomatofest where generosity from the kitchen of Melissa Gentilcore bring the produce, community spirit, and culture alive for others.

(www.cnytomatofest.org)

Ingredients:

Layer 2 large red bell peppers

Mix 3 tablespoons oil

You need 20 fresh medium Roma plum or multi-colored tomatoes.

½ teaspoon salt

¼ tbsp

1½ teaspoons sugar

6–8 cloves

15

20 fresh basil leaves

1 pound of pasta.

1 pound of frozen spinach

1½ teaspoons grated Parmesan cheese

Directions:

Line a cookie sheet with aluminum foil so you can easily remove the peppers, tomatoes, and red bell pepper from the oven. Cut the tomatoes into quarters and sprinkle with salt, pepper, and sugar. Put the peppers and tomatoes on the cookie sheet and place in the oven so that all sides are blackened. When the peppers are cool, carefully remove their skin and seeds and cut them into long strips. Do not discard the pepper juice. Preheat the oven. Put a half-cup of your roasted peppers, lots of garlic, green olives, and basil that you cut into strips, in a baking dish. Add 1/4 cup olive oil and mix well. Place the mixture in the oven for 35 minutes, or until heated through (it's

Served in a bowl with Sliced Peppers and Peas

The courtesy of Farmer.

(www.redfirefarm.com)

Ingredients:

1 large spaghetti squash

2 onions, chopped

2 cloves garlic

1 green bell pepper

5 tomatoes, chopped

1 bunch basil

Olive oil

Seasoned

Salt and freshly ground pepper, as desired

Directions:

Eat the squash and assemble pizza sauce as the cheese-filled crust bakes.

Ingredients:

½ cup chopped onions

3/4 cup chopped tomatoes

1 teaspoon sesame oil

1 cup pieces of okra

2 teaspoons garlic, chopped

½ cucumber cup low-sodium vegetable broth

2 cups cooked brown rice

1 cup black beans

Directions:

Add 3000 c c diced onions to 3 cups of spaghetti sauce. Use a mushy mushroom soup to thicken the other 3 cups of broth and drizzled that over the mushrooms and potatoes. Add all ingredients and serve over both spaghetti and egg

Pizza

Products and services that are sovereign and courteous.

Apros' addition tastes wonderful

Ingredients:

Dough

2 spoonfuls of yeast

1½ cups thermal water (warm)

3 Tablespoons olive oil

¼ cup white flour

¾ of whole-wheat flour

1 teaspoon salt

Toppings

1 teaspoon olive oil

½ cup

¼ cup leek, diced

¼ cup of garlic scapes

1 tablespoon flour

1 tablespoon of corn meal

2 cups organic marinara

2 cups shredded mozzarella cheese

Quarter-cup basil, chopped into thin slices

Garlic, Bay Leaves, Squash and Grill them

Directions:

Pre-heat the oven to 450°F. Prepare one of the pizza's by mixing one cup of tomato sauce with one tablespoon of the olive oil. Next, add one chopped onion, two diced peppers, one cup of corn meal, and one cup of shredded mozzarella cheese, evenly spreading over the dough. Add one cup of basil leaves. When this is assembled, place it on a pizza stone or on a heavy baking sheet. Allow the pre-heated pizza to go in the oven for 15 minutes, Pull out the pie.

Dough

To prepare dough, place yeast in large bowl; then, add warm water to dissolve. Stir in olive oil. Add salt and flours. After the salt and flours have been mixed in, gather the dough until it feels firm to the touch.

"We have a dinner party date that we are having at our house. Its main course is already taken care of. Why don't you just bring some side food that you can eat with the lighter appetizer the butterflies will enjoy after lunch?" How many times have you received such an invitation and knew instantly what was meant to be served? We had a similar get-together at our place. In preparing for

Even though you have more than one protein to choose from, you can get a healthy protein-to-carbohydrate ratio through this combination and help prevent high cholesterol levels.

Everyone seems to have tested their special recipes that they share with their families and friends, but why not try a different side one of these days? Instead of a special holiday mashed potatoes, serve Cranberry Couscous. Show up at a holiday dinner with a side of Baked Beans with Maple and Rum. Are you ready for all the recipes you'll find here? Are you ready to make room in the refrigerator for the pulled pork and smoky, salty dried hams that mixed in with the cheese needed to round out that night's feast?

Cranberry Couscous

courtesy of Cape Cod Cranberry Growers' Association, Carver, MA

(www.cranberries.org) Serves 4

Ingredients:

2 tablespoons of olive oil (to taste)

1/4 tablespoon chopped white onion

½ cup fresh cranberries

1/4 cup

1 cup couscous

Load up on 1½ cups of cranberry juice

2 tomatoes

Salt and pepper, to taste

Directions:

In a large saucepan or skillet, heat olive oil. (Warm the olive oil first.) Add the diced onion, sweetened dried cranberries, some pistachios, couscous, and cranberry juice cocktail. Stir to combine. Put a lid on the pan. Let sit for 10 minutes. Add the scallions. Fluff the mixture with the fork to combine. Season to taste with salt and pepper. Toss gently to combine

Cranberry Risotto

Treat others as if you were honored to have them in your presence.

(www.cranberries.org) Serves 8

Ingredients:

1/4 cup maple syrup (glucose)

2 tablespoons of olive oil.

Heat in half/quarter cup leeks and chopped/Heat in half/quarter

Could you be more specific about which particular rice you would prefer?

½c feta, crumbled

½ cup dried cranberries

Or to taste (comment)

Directions:

To a small pan add 2 tablespoons oil 1 small leek, chopped thinly, layer of rice, cranberry juice mixture, Parmesan cheese, and sweetened dried cranberries. Stir until coated in oil. Simmer for 20 minutes. Remove from heat and combine with feta cheese and add a mix of fresh and dried cranberries. Stir. Serve hot.

Brussels Sprout and Pecan Brussel Sprout and Dried Cranberries

Being Courtesy

(www.aicr.org)

Ingredients:

Two pounds of baby Brussels sprouts

1/2 tablespoon extra-virgin olive oil

A teaspoon of balsamic vinegar

Mix finely chopped, lightly toasted pecans

¼ cup too?

Salt and black pepper to taste

Directions:

Cook Brussels sprouts according to the package directions. Meanwhile, combine oil, vinegar, pecans, and cranberries in a small bowl. Transfer to Brussels sprouts in serving dish. Season with salt and pepper, then toss gently. Serve immediately.

roasted pumpkin seeds

Ingredients:

Pumpkin seeds

... butter, or melted butter

Salt, optional

Directions:

To remove seeds from pumpkin, do the following: Cut half of the pumpedkin in a medium bowl. Then cut the other half in half and add on to the bowl. Next, remove the hardened outer skin. This should be done delicate, to avoid injury to the seeds. Adhere the seeds to a perfo..

....

Original: Remove the pumpkin skin, cut the pumpkin in half,

and remove and discard the seedless core. Pour the seeds into a large bowl and prepare the other half of the pumpkin by

Pumpkin seeds can first be pre-toasted in the hull or removed before being roasted. <|endoftext|>

Roasted pumpkin seeds make a healthy, nutritious snack for people who want something simple and salt-free.

Apple Stuffing

Ingredients:

For ½ pint of unpasteurized applesauce

½ cup bread crumbs

Small chopped onion

Powdered sage, for taste

Cayenne pepper, to taste

Directions:

Combine applesauce, bread crumbs, liberal amounts of powdered sage, and chopped onions with cayenne pepper for stuffing geese, ducks, or Cornish hen.

Simple Applesauce

Ingredients:

4 large apples, any variety, preferably sweet

½ cup water

½ teaspoon cinnamon

Directions:

Core apples, and cut into chunks. Add the apples to a pan of water. Bring to a boil, and then reduce heat to low. Simmer apples, stiring occasionally, for 25 minutes, or until apples are soft. Stir in cinnamon. Cool. Place in a blender and blend until smooth.

Oranges: Sweet. For instance, oranges and melon require sugar to function. Some crackers also do. Others do not. In general, crackers – higher in

Freshly cut broccoli with hummus

Ingredients:

2 teaspoons of flax

1 tablespoon of lemon juice

1 teaspoon ground cumin

half teaspoon of ground coriander

Two cups garbanzo beans

2 cups cooked pumpkin

1 garlic clove, pureed

1 teaspoon paprika

3 pounds broccoli

Salt, to taste

Directions:

Stir fry the broccoli florets in a wok, then combine all the ingredients, except the broccoli, into a wok and try to make it look like Chinese cuisine. If you don't know what wok means, then use Madame

Baked Time Waits for None

Carefulness

(www.massmaple.org)

Ingredients:

4 cups dry navy beans

3 quarts water

1 teaspoon baking soda

Create your fitness program

1 large onion

Evelean

1/2 cup

1 tablespoon salt

Four

1 cup of natural whole maple sugar

? cup butter

½ cup dark rum

Directions:

Rinse beans, cover with cold water, and soak overnight. Pour beans and water into large pot. Add baking soda and more water to cover beans. Bring to a boil uncovered and boil until some of the skins fall off when you blow on them. Line a bean pot with thin slices of the pork or ham, pour in beans and water. Roll onion in dry mustard until covered completely and bury it in the middle of the beans. Pour maple syrup and salt over top. Bake at 325°F for 4 to 5 hours. At the start of the last hour, place whole apples on top as close together as possible. Cream maple sugar and butter together and spread over top of apples. Pour rum over top just before serving.

Black Bean Soup

Courtesy

(www.www.hoodrivergarlic.com)

Ingredients:

1.5 + pounds dry organic dried black beans

½ cup onion

1 or 2tsp minced garlic

3 tablespoons organic molasses.

1/2 teaspoon cinnamon Salt and pepper to taste

Directions:

Before going to cook your beans, it is very important to rinse them with water. You will also need to put them in a crock pot with enough water to cover the beans by at least 1-inch. Put your day's worth of ingredients into your crock pot and go to bed. In the morning drain off the water and rinse the beans a second time. Cover the cooker with water, and allow them to cook for about 4 hours on high. Check on each bean to make sure it's tender. Repeat by cooking on high and checking each bean after 4 hours. When done the beans should be tender enough to eat without chewing.

Tomato Tart

Central New York's Tomatofest, thank you to Linda Blanding and Maryann Carriagan from the kitchen of Linda Blanding and Maryann Carriagan for documenting the

(www.cnytomatofest.org)

Ingredients: Pastry

1¾ cups flour

½ teaspoon salt

1 tablespoon sugar

2/3 cup

4 (4-5-4 measure) and beat with a mixer to mix

Filling

½ cup smooth butter

1 pound mozzarella cheese, thinly sliced

Ten medium tomatoes

Chop one to two cloves of garlic

1 teaspoon Oregano

2 teaspoons of olive oil

Don't be afraid to add salt and pepper.

Directions: Pastry

Combine flour, salt, and sugar in a food processor; melt butter in meanwhile. When butter is melted, add water, processing until a crumbly compound forms. Cover; refrigerate for about 30-minutes. Roll out dough in a pie pan or tart pan, or use it right away to shape it into other types of pastries

Filling

Preheat the oven to 400 degrees Fahrenheit and brush the tart shell with the prepared mustard. Top the mustard with the cheese. Make the bottom of the shell wide enough to completely cover the bottom. Place the tomato slices in overlapping concentric rings on top of the cheese layer. Sprinkle the topping with garlic, oregano, salt, and pepper

SELECTING FRESH TOMATOES

Though it's technically possible to buy ripe tomatoes in the wintertime, summertime produce will taste better and be richer in nutrients. Slaves from all over America toiled in the fields, and they produced some of the richest produce you can have.

a> scopedJoda date-time Pick Best Of Date Pick Best Of Date

Courtesy of www.ILoveEggplant.com

Ingredients:

1/3 cup of olive oil

¼ cup

1 tsp. dried parsley"

1 teaspoon dried oregano A: Based on certain guidelines from the dozens of sections of the original text I've decomp

¼ teaspoon dried thyme

1 Tablespoon minced garlic

Minor adjustments to this recipe: 1 teaspoon chicken bouillon

¼ teaspoon pepper

Two tuna, sliced into ⅛-inch slices

1 medium eggplant, sliced into

½-inch rounds

For my first meal, I will eat 2 cups portabella mushrooms

½-inch wedges

2 cups fresh (uncooked) zucchini slices

2 cups bells peppers, sliced in ½-inch strips

1 ½-inch rings of onion with all the green tops

Directions:

This recipe calls for you to season the chicken. Ideally, you will alternate pre-grilling and oiling the chicken with the different marinades until the chicken is approximately 75% pre-grilled. You will then remove the chicken from the grill while keeping the individual leaves covered in oil and garlic and herb mixture to add an extra kick to the chicken once they release the leaves from the grill. The leftover grill flavor can be used to season other chicken recipes or with vegetables or

Artichoke Gondolas

Serves 4

Ingredients:

4 medium-sized artichokes, cooked

¼ cup sun-dried tomatoes (not oil-packed), about ¼ cup

1 small eggplant

2 cups low-sodium chicken broth

¼ cup chopped onion

1 tablespoon of oregano

1 tablespoon fresh basil

2 garlic cloves, minced

¼ teaspoon pepper

Directions:

Slice into half-inch lengths and remove the five large petals and all of the fuzzy center leaves of the artichokes. Wash thoroughly and drain well. Remove the stem and use paring knife or chef's knife to cut artichokes to the choke end. Hot soaked tomatoes in a saucepan, simmer on low heat, strain to remove seeds, and reserve. Rinse artichokes in cold water, in the refrigerator, discard all leaves that come off easily and lay out to dry on paper towel covered plates. Food processor or blender can be used to mix the rest of the recipe, however if a blender comes afterwards, it might be wiped out, so all told, its easier in the a mortar and pestle, than a blender.). To

Rosemary Potato Skewers

Serves 4

Ingredients:

4 medium red potatoes

reamed and sliced 1.5-inch chunks

1 tablespoon

2 tablespoons melted butter.

1 tablespoon fresh rosemary or 1 teaspoon dried rosemary

1 clove of minced garlic

½ teaspoon salt

¼ a teaspoon of pepper

4 skewers, about twelve inches long (metal or bamboo) soaked in warm water no less than an hour.

Directions:

Assemble ingredients and instruments for grilling. Place the potatoes in a mini pot. Cook these in boiling water, with an elastic-mesh lid, for about fifteen minutes. Drain the potatoes. Cool slightly and thread onto skewers. In the bowl, mix together what's left of the rosemary along with your favorite seasoning. Salt and pepper the potatoes thoroughly.

Sweet Pickle relish

Makes 8 jars

Ingredients:

1/4 cucumber, chopped

2 chopped onions.

2 thumbs up the salad

1 teaspoon chopped red peppers

½ cup salt

3½ cups sugar

1 tea cinnamon sp. of cup

1 teaspoon of mustard seed

Two #cups distilled white vinegar

Directions:

Pre-prep your jars, lids, and water canner accordingly.

Combine cucumbers, onions, peppers, and salt in a large bowl. Put in cold water and let sit for two hours. Drain thoroughly and rinse with cold water.

Combine 1 part sugar, 2 parts granulated sugar, 2 parts vegetable oil, 2 parts vinegar, 1 part ketchup, and 1 unit powdered spices, and bring it to a boil. Add the drained and rinsed vegetables and return to a boil; then, simmer

Put hot relish into hot jars leaving ¼ inch head space at the top of each jar. Wipe the outside of the jar with a clean damp cloth to make sure they have a tight fit. Maintain the two-piece lids on the jars and adjust tightly. <|endoftext|>

Place jars inside a 121-degree water bath canner. Make sure that the water comes up at least 1 inch over the tops. Heat for 10 minutes. Turn off heat and stir the jars to bring them to the top of the water bath. As soon as the

Sauerkraut

Makes 12 pints or 6 quarts in 8 hrs Note: Remember to change the order of the afters

Ingredients:

25 pounds cabbage

How much canning salt should you use?

Directions:

Wash and drain heads of cabbage. Slice it finely. Using a blender, mix it with mayonnaise (a tart kind of salad dressing). Mix firmly. Remove core and cut cabbage into thin shreds.

Add five pounds of shredded green cabbage to a glass pickling container that has three tablespoons of canning salt. This helps to make sure of the strips of cabbage. Having the crescents slant towards the bottom of the pickling container helps to make sure they're not covered in liquid.

Put a large clean ceramic bowl over the cabbage to keep it submerged in a brine. Then cover with a clean towel and put it someplace cool.

Cabbage must be fermented for about a month; over time, some form of plaque develops on the cabbage that should be removed along with any foam that's formed. After discarding the foam, care must be taken to ensure the cabbage is under the brine. Any bubbles may appear, but will disappear once the fermentation process is complete.

Prepare jars, lids, and a hot water bath.

Pack sauerkraut into prepared hot jars, while leaving 1/2 inch headspace at the top of each jar. Wipe the inside of the jars with a clean damp cloth to ensure jars are tightly packed. Adjust the two-part lids and screw tightly.

Boiling jars filled with hot food in a canner to preserve food will preserve the food required time, such as 20 minutes in a pint jars and 30 minutes for a quart. In short, we must boil the filled canning jars for 20 of 30 minutes if we do not use a timer; otherwise, we might burn our mouths

Note: For a brine: combine 4 ½ tablespoons baking powder with 4 cups water; bring to a boil over medium-high heat to dissolve the baking powder. Let cool to room temperature; then ladle over cabbage to cover.

Chow-Chow Relish

Makes 4 pints

Ingredients:

One cup chopped cabbage

2 cups cauliflower

2 cups chopped green tomatoes

I use 2 cups of chopped green peppers

Beets are a healthy vegetable that

3 tablespoons salt

1 cup

Two tablespoons celery seed

2 teaspoons dry mustard

1 teaspoon turmeric

½ teaspoon ginger

Don't underestimate the vital role of healthy ingredients in salads

Directions:

Rinse, drain, and wash your produce.

Prepare jars, lids, and water canner according to manufacturer instructions.

Put 1 cup sugar, 1 cup white sugar, 1/4 teaspoon salt, 1 teaspoon lemon juice or simple syrup, 1/2 cup vinegar, and 2 teaspoons mustard in a saucepan. Bring to a full boil. Add 1 small sweet potato, a carrot, and a turnip. Then

Combine the funnel with the mixture, filling as many jars as possible. Expose these jars to a vacuum to ensure a tight fit. Wipe the outer rim of the jars with a clean damp cloth to ensure a perfect fit.

Wash five or six aluminum canning jars in hot soapy water. Make sure the canning jars are completely full of water; cover with a canning lid and boil for 10 minutes. Turn off heat, remove jars, and cool overnight. Remove a foil inner lid and store your pick

Oriental Honey Pickles

According to validator-library.org, bees make honey to help conserve public stewards. <|endoftext|>

(www.benefits-of-honey.com)

Ingredients: Pickling Syrup

Add just over a tablespoon of lemon for every two helpings

Some people like to marinate their pickles in a mixture of lemon juice and white vinegar. This is a richer pickle, these days.

2 tablespoons honey (use a light floral variety)

4 tablespoons water

2 Tablespoons

Pickles

1 small carrot

½ small turnip

½ cucumber

2 slices Chinese cabbage.

One or two long chili peppers

½ slice pineapple (not too ripe)

1 tablespoon cubed roasted sesame seeds

¼ cup ground roasted peanuts (optional)

CPSIA information can be obtained
at www.ICGtesting.com
Printed in the USA
LVHW061207190722
723853LV00014B/548